THIS BOOK should find a place in every home where young children ask, "How are babies born?"

Written by a doctor and his wife who are authorities in the fields of child psychology and sex education, it has been approved by representatives of the Catholic, Protestant, and Jewish clergy and tested with a group of children. Educators and child guidance groups will find this book a valuable aid in their work with children from six to ten.

But this is a book for parents to read to a child; a book for the child to read himself. Here he will find the story of how life begins told objectively and with dignity. Facts are presented simply and directly. And, without being sentimental, there is an emphasis on family love.

A BABY IS BORN

A Baby Is Born

The Story of How Life Begins

By MILTON I. LEVINE, M.D.
Clinical Professor of Pediatrics, Cornell University-New York Hospital Medical Center

and JEAN H. SELIGMANN
Formerly Assistant Nursery School Teacher, Bank Street Schools, New York City

Illustrations by J. WILLIAM MYERS

Revised Edition

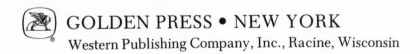 GOLDEN PRESS • NEW YORK
Western Publishing Company, Inc., Racine, Wisconsin

ACKNOWLEDGMENTS

The authors wish to express their appreciation and gratitude to all those who advised in the preparation of this book. Especially do we wish to thank for their helpful advice and criticism members of the Department of Pediatrics, Cornell University Medical College; members of the staff of the Child Study Association of America; Dr. Milton J. E. Senn, Emeritus Sterling Professor of Pediatrics and Psychiatry, Yale University; Mrs. Eleanor Brussel, Director of Nursery Education, Horace Mann School, New York City; Dr. Anita Bell, Children's Psychoanalyst; Dr. Robert Simonds, Psychoanalyst; as well as representatives of the Catholic, Protestant and Jewish clergy; and of special importance, a number of children whose advice was invaluable.

To Carol and Ann

Contents

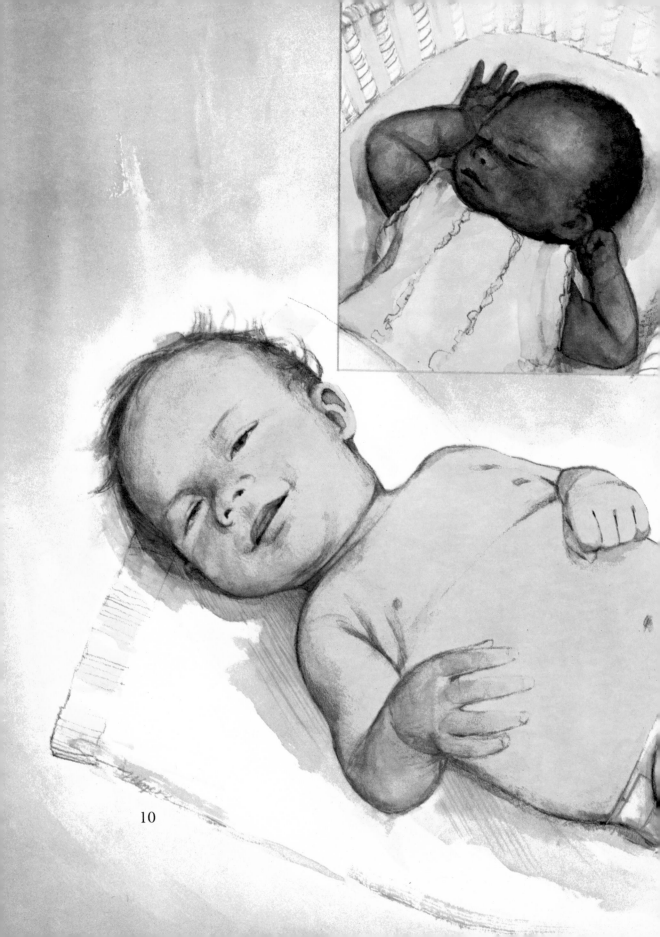

10

When You Were a Baby

Have you ever seen pictures of yourself when you were just a tiny baby? You looked very different from the way you do now, didn't you? You probably had little or no hair on your head, no teeth in your mouth. You could not walk or talk when you were that little, either. All you could do when you wanted something was cry, and to get from one place to another you had to be carried.

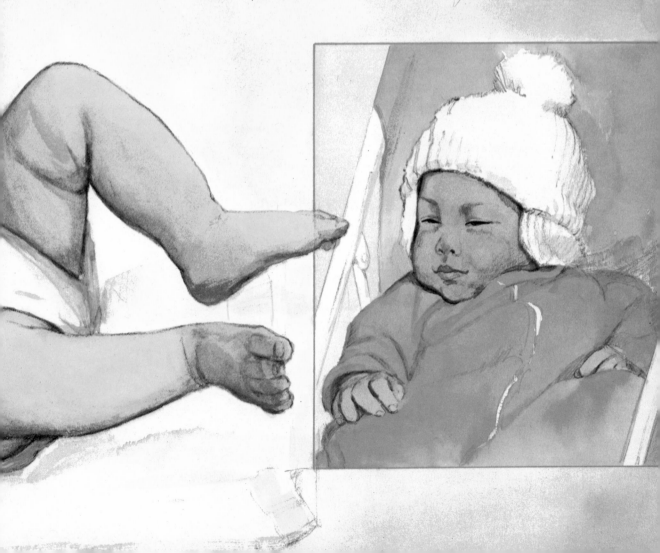

But gradually you grew up, you learned to walk and talk and sing, to run and jump and play. You had to do quite a lot of growing and changing before you came to be the way you are now. But have you ever wondered how you became alive, how you were born, how you really came to be a living baby? You had to grow and change a good deal, too, while you were becoming a baby — and here is the story of how all that happens.

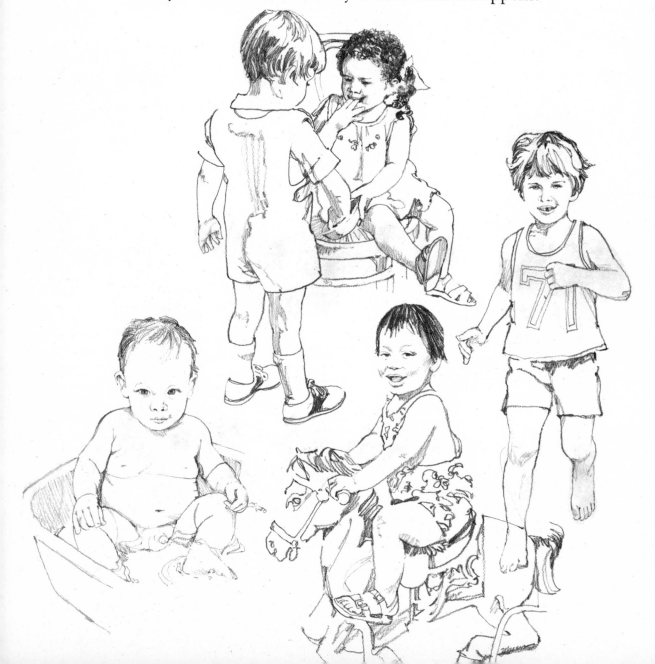

Where Did You Come From?

You began your life as a tiny egg that was inside your mother's body. This egg was not at all like a chicken's egg. It was not like any egg that you have ever seen but was just a tiny speck of an egg, even smaller than one tiny little grain of salt. You would have to have extremely sharp eyes to be able to see this kind of egg.

The egg is even smaller than the dot at the end of this sentence. If it were very, very much larger, it would look like a round ball, something like this—

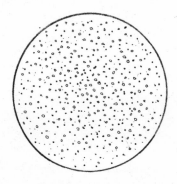

It is hard to believe that huge animals like the elephant, and tiny insects like the ant, all began in the same way from a tiny egg. And isn't it exciting to think that this person that is you, your body and arms and legs and head, all started out as something so small that it could scarcely be seen?

Practically every animal that you know about began its life as an egg—every fish, frog, ant, fly, beetle, bird, cat, dog, even monkeys, elephants, giraffes, crocodiles, lions, tigers — yes, almost every animal that you could mention.

Every animal has babies of the same kind as the mother and father animal.

A mother and father cow have baby cows—calves—for their babies. A mother and father cat have baby cats—kittens—for their babies. A mother and a father horse have baby horses—foals—for their babies.

People like your father and your mother are called human beings, and human beings have human babies which grow up to be children—boys and girls—just like you.

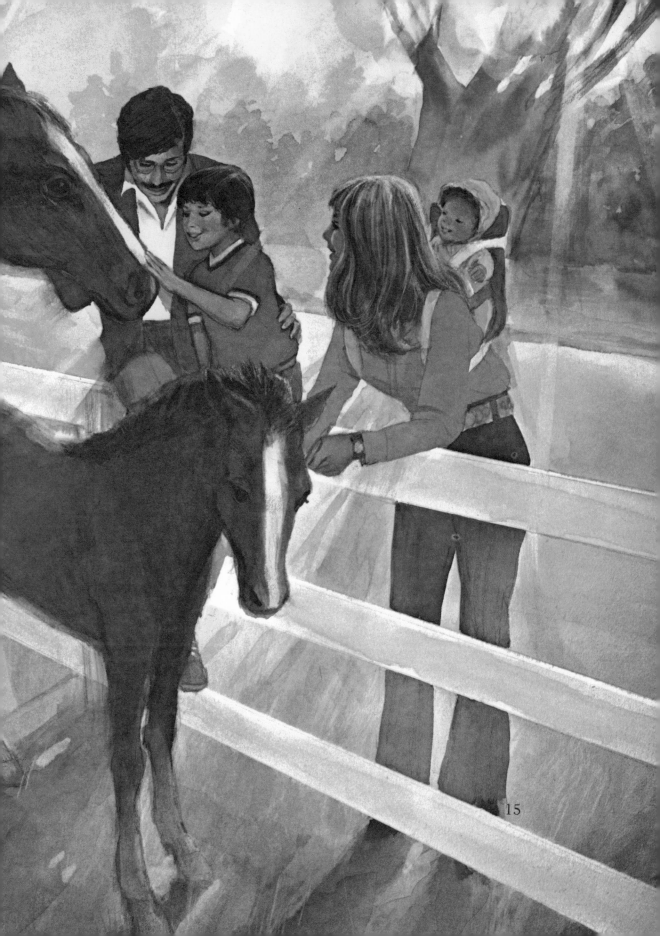

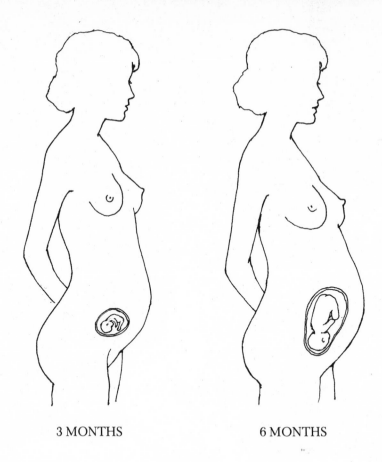

3 MONTHS   6 MONTHS

Where Does the Egg Grow To Be a Baby?

We said that every baby animal and every human baby starts from an egg. In human beings this egg grows to be a baby inside the mother's body in a place below the stomach. This place is called the *uterus* or *womb*. The uterus is hollow, and is shaped something like a pear. It is about the size of a medium-sized pear, too.

In the mother's uterus a wonderful thing happens. The tiny egg grows and grows and changes until finally, after quite a long time—about nine months—it has grown and

16

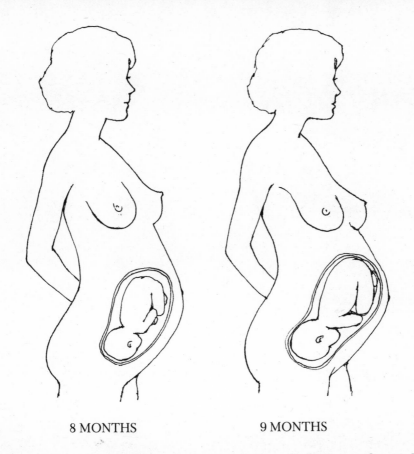

8 MONTHS   9 MONTHS

changed and developed into a living baby, ready to be born.

Almost every part of the body does its own work: the heart pumps the blood, the stomach digests the food that you eat, the eyes see, the ears hear. The uterus—which is only in the woman's body and never in the man's—is where babies live and grow before they are born. And so every human baby begins its life in its mother's uterus, which is the special part of the mother's body just for babies.

A special tube or passage called the *vagina* leads from the uterus to the outside of the mother's body. The opening of the vagina on the outside of the body is between the legs, just behind the opening for urine.

17

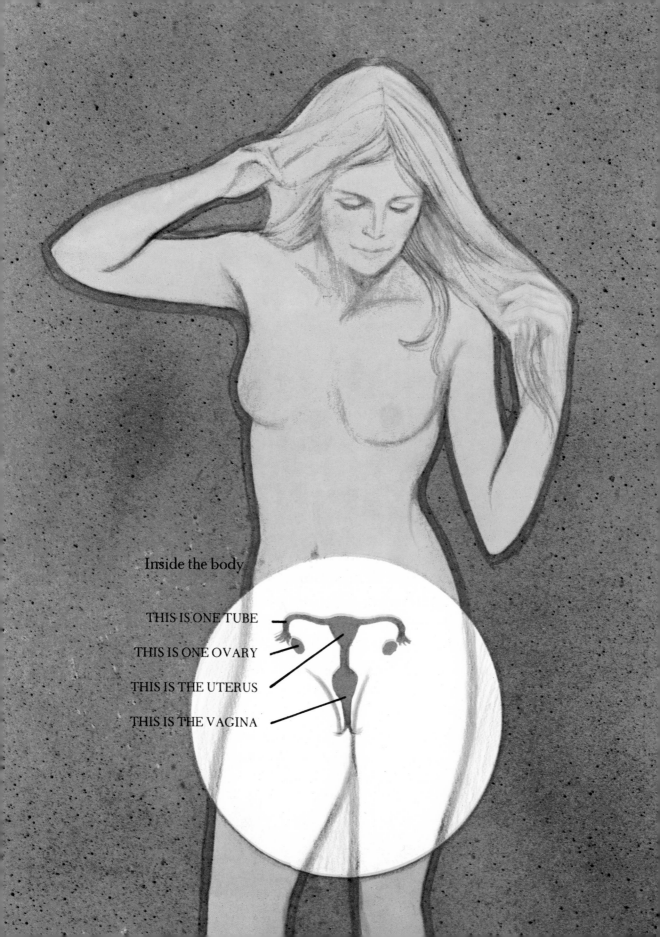

Inside the body

THIS IS ONE TUBE

THIS IS ONE OVARY

THIS IS THE UTERUS

THIS IS THE VAGINA

Where Does the Egg Come From?

Almost all she-animals — we call them female animals—have hundreds of eggs inside their bodies. Women, too, have hundreds of eggs inside their bodies. They are in two small parts of the body on each side of the uterus. These parts of the body are called the *ovaries*. The ovaries are flat and oval in shape. They are about the size and shape of almond nuts.

Right next to each ovary is a tube which goes into the uterus. Once every month, in grown-up girls and women, a single egg comes out of one ovary or the other, and travels down this tube into the uterus. That is how the egg, which will grow to be a baby, gets into the uterus.

The eggs that do not grow to be babies—and many, many do not—just pass into the uterus where they break up and can no longer be seen.

What Makes the Egg Grow into a Baby?

The little egg cannot grow to be a baby all by itself. Something has to join with it in order to make it the kind of egg which will develop into a baby. This something is called a *sperm*, and it comes from the body of the father.

A sperm is also very, very tiny, much tinier than the egg. Not even the sharpest eyes can see a sperm. It can be seen only through a microscope. A microscope is like a very strong magnifying glass. It makes everything look much larger. Through it a sperm looks like a little tadpole or polliwog—an oval body with a long, thin, wiggling tail.

This is the way a sperm looks if you see it through a microscope—

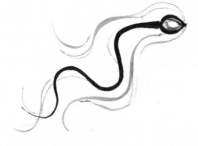

Like a tadpole, the sperm swims about and moves by quickly wiggling its tail.

The sperm is in the father. The egg is in the mother. No egg in the mother can grow to be a baby by itself. It can grow into a baby only if a sperm joins with it. This means that the sperm has to leave the father's body and meet the egg inside the mother's body. This means, too, that there has to be a mother and a father to make a baby. That is why you might look like your father even though you grew inside your mother. Something from your mother—the egg—and something from your father—the sperm—joined together to make you.

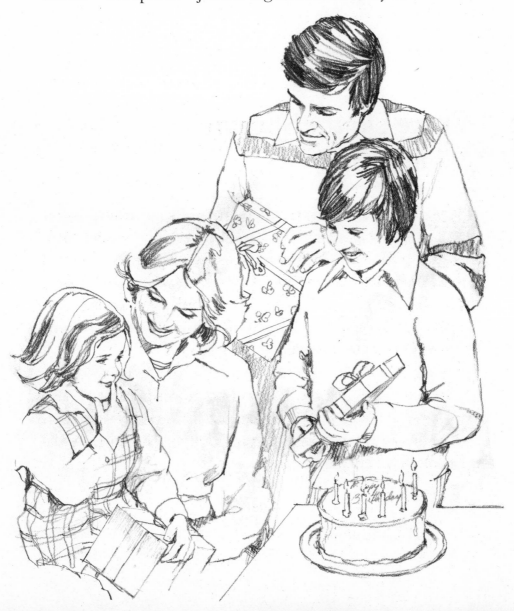

Where Do the Sperms Come From?

Most he-animals—we call them *male* animals—have many millions of sperms in their bodies. The sperms are made in two small parts of the body called *testicles*. In many male animals, such as male horses, cats, dogs, monkeys, goats, pigs, sheep, and bulls, the testicles are inside a loose bag, or sac, of skin which hangs between the hind legs on the outside of the body.

Boys and men have testicles, too. In men the testicles are oval-shaped and are about the size of walnuts. They also are in a sac of skin which hangs between the legs on the outside of the body. And it is in these testicles that all the millions of sperms are made.

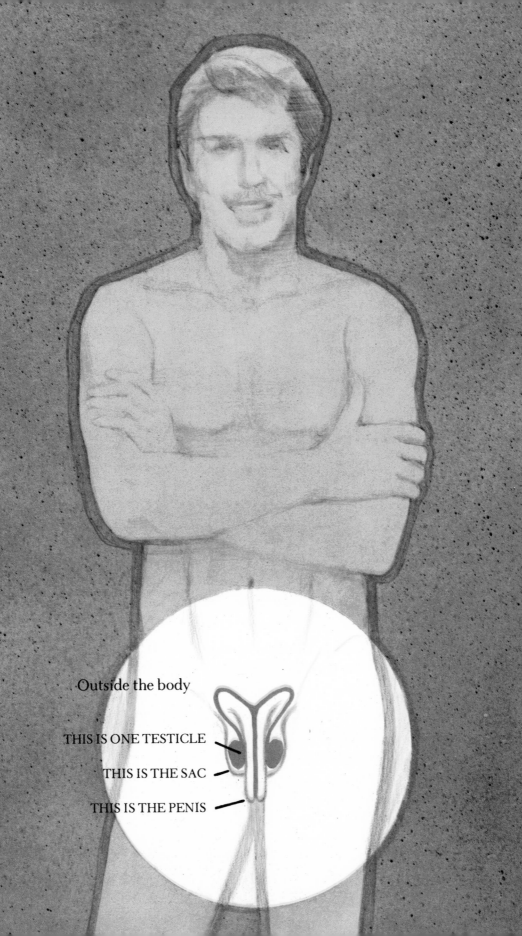

Outside the body

THIS IS ONE TESTICLE

THIS IS THE SAC

THIS IS THE PENIS

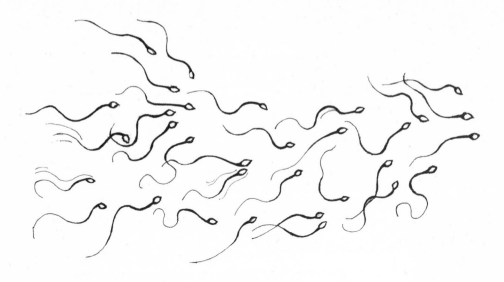

How Do the Sperms Get Out of the Body?

In front of the sac which holds the testicles is a part of the body shaped something like a thumb. This is called the *penis*. Only male animals, and boys and men, have a penis and testicles. You probably know that inside the penis is a tube through which urine comes out of the body. But the penis has another use, too. It is through the same tube in the penis that the sperms pass out of the body. Here is an interesting thing, though: the sperms and the urine cannot pass through this tube at the same time.

Sperms must have some liquid in which to swim. The testicles help to make a white liquid, which is known as *semen*. The sperms, swimming around in this special liquid, leave the body of the male through the penis.

How Does the Sperm
Get to the Egg?

You already know that practically every animal started as an egg that had been joined by a sperm. But the way in which the sperm meets the egg is different in different animals.

A mother fish, for example, lays many eggs in the water. The father fish comes along and pours his sperms over these eggs from an opening on the underside of his body near his tail. Just some of the eggs are reached and joined by the sperms, and only those eggs that have been joined by sperms will grow to be baby fishes.

What about frogs? A mother frog also lays many hundreds of eggs at one time. But, before she lays them, the father frog gets on her back, and as the eggs leave the body of the mother, he pours his sperms over them.

Once again, only those eggs that are reached and joined by sperms will develop into tadpoles, which later become frogs.

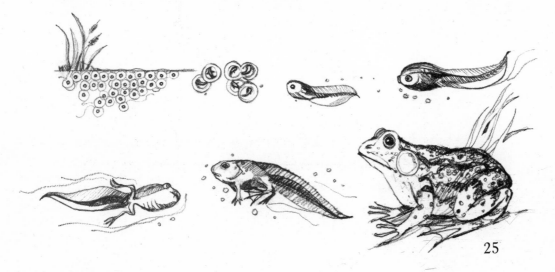

With frogs and fishes, the sperms enter the eggs *outside* the bodies of the mother animals. In many other animals such as insects, birds, horses, dogs, cats, lions, tigers, and also human beings, the sperms and eggs join together *inside* of the mother's body.

How do the sperms of the rooster meet the eggs of the hen? A rooster gets on to the back of the hen. The sperms come out of an opening under his tail feathers and enter the hen's body through an opening under her tail feathers. This opening leads to the place *inside* of the hen where the eggs are stored. The sperms swim to the eggs, and here some of the sperms enter and join with the eggs. Only one sperm can enter an egg. Then a hard shell forms over each egg. The hen lays these eggs, sits on them, keeping them warm, and baby chicks hatch from each egg that was joined by a sperm.

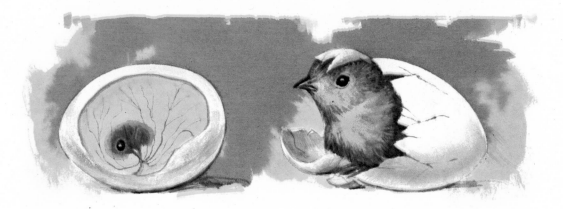

Hens lay eggs even if the eggs have not been joined by sperms. But, of course, these eggs will never grow to be baby chicks. In fact, these are the eggs that you usually eat.

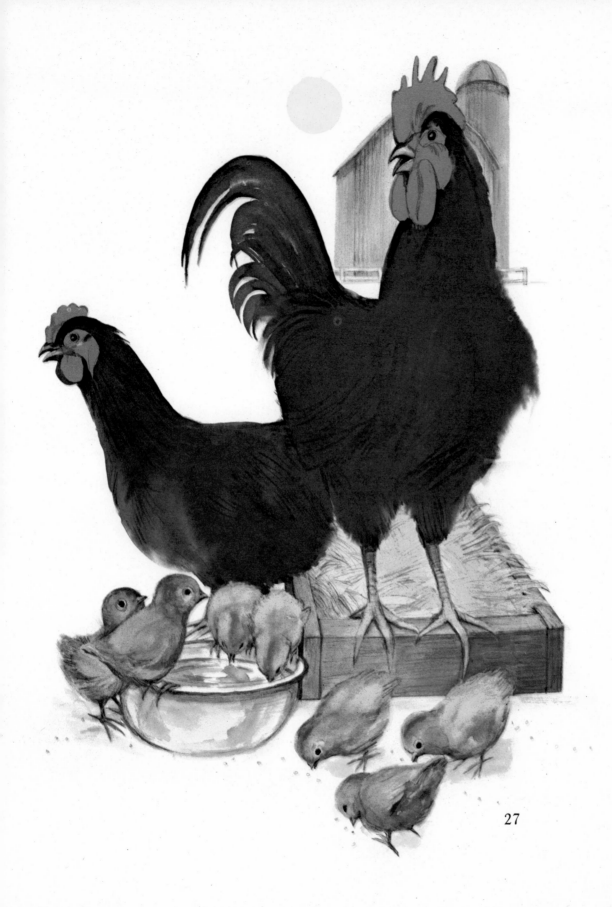

27

In cows, also, the sperm joins the egg inside the mother's body. The bull, like many other male animals, has a penis on the under part of his body near the hind legs. When mating with the cow, the bull mounts upon the rear part of the cow's body. The penis then slips into the opening (the vagina) between the back legs of the cow. Through the penis the sperms go from the bull to the cow. The sperms, once they have entered the vagina of the cow, swim up the vagina to the place inside the cow where the egg is. With cows—as with human beings and as with some other animals—there is usually only one egg ready at a time. After the sperm has joined with the egg, this egg will grow and change and develop, until it grows to be a baby cow—a calf.

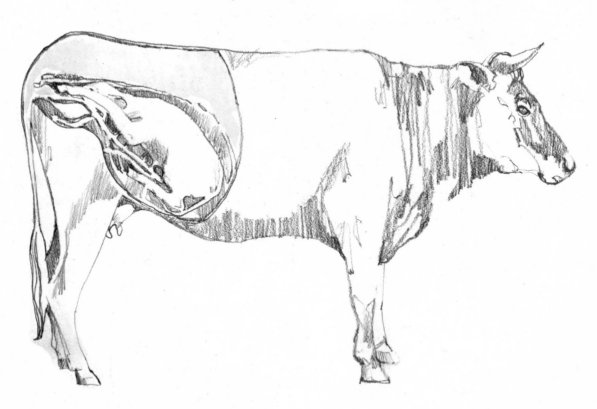

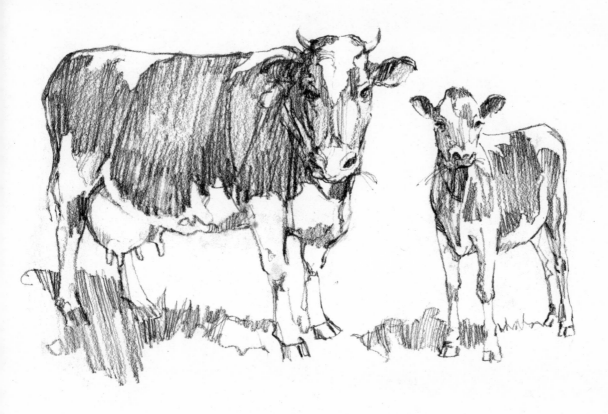

The mother cow does not lay her eggs the way the mother hen does. Instead, the baby calf develops *inside* the mother's body, in the uterus. After a certain time, the mother gives birth to the baby calf out of the same opening through which the sperms entered—that is, the vagina.

Human babies are made in about the same way.

This is how it happens. The father and the mother lie close together, and the penis enters the vagina. The sperms, in the semen, then pass out of the father's penis and swim up into the uterus of the mother and from there into the tubes, where an egg might be waiting.

Mothers and Fathers

There are many differences between human and other animal parents. Among animals, such as dogs and cats and cows and horses, the father chooses any female animal for his mate. Almost any female will do as long as she is the same kind of animal he is. Dogs mate with dogs, pigs with pigs, goats with goats, horses with horses. With most animals, the father and the mother do not even stay together—and if they do, it is only for a very short time.

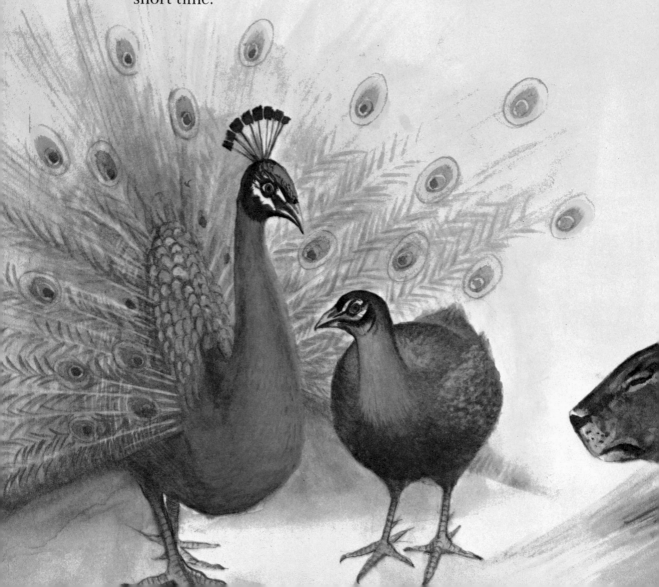

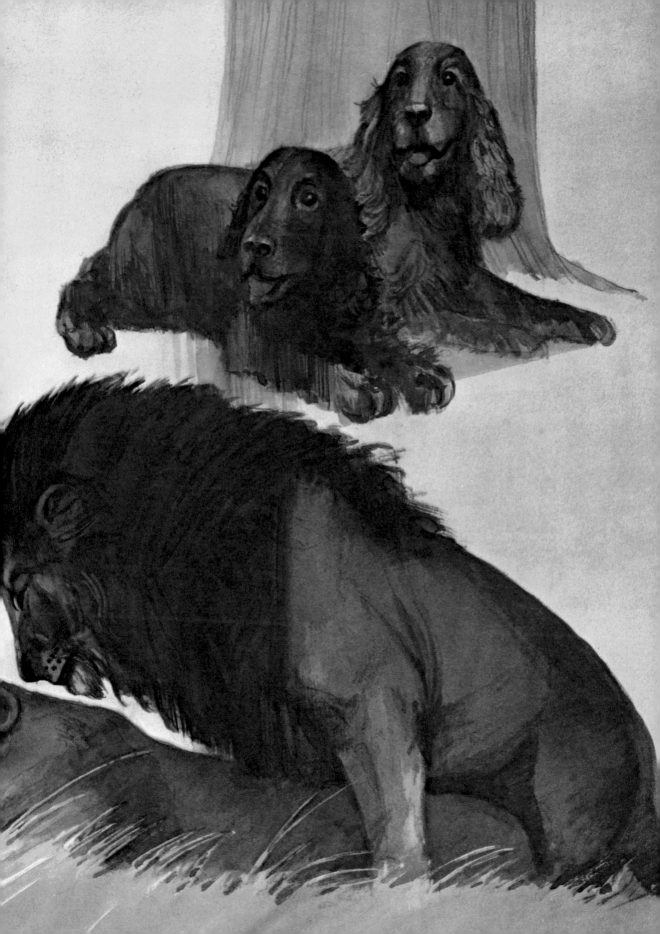

But men and women usually choose their mates with great care and try to know each other quite well before they decide to be married. And if they really love one another, they will want to get married, to have a home, to have children, and to live together for the rest of their lives.

Men and women show how much they love each other in many ways. They show it by being very happy with one another, by kissing, by hugging, by wanting children, and by having children whom they can love together.

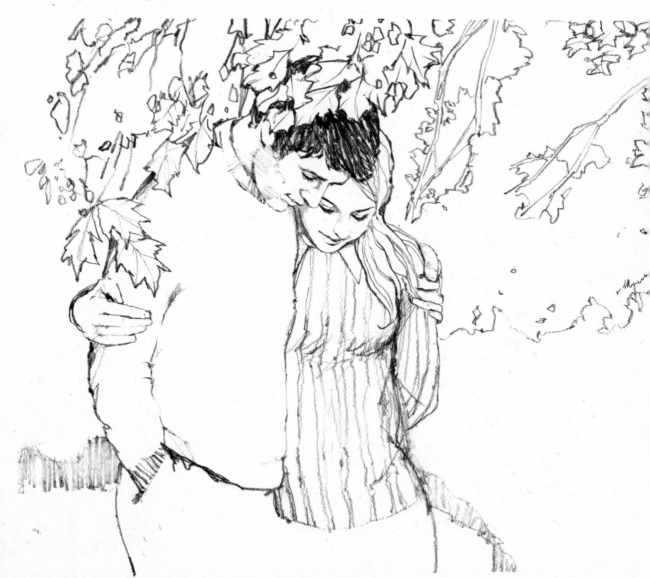

After the Sperm
Has Joined With the Egg

You remember that in women, about once a month, an egg comes down the tube that leads from the ovary to the uterus. When the sperms from the father enter the vagina, many sperms swim up into the tube where the egg is. But of these millions of sperms, strangely enough, usually only *one* can enter an egg. The rest of the sperms soon are passed out of her body through the vagina. The single sperm enters the egg and becomes part of it. There are no longer a separate egg and sperm. These two are now one and form what is called a *fertilized* egg. It is only from fertilized eggs that babies can grow.

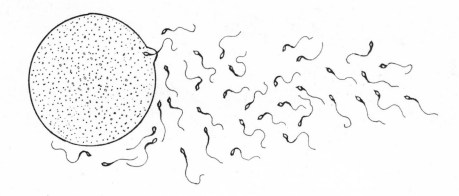

The fertilized egg continues its journey in the tube and enters the uterus. Then it becomes attached to the inside lining of the uterus, and begins to grow. It's hard to believe, but in nine months this tiny little egg, which has been joined with an even tinier sperm, will grow to be a living human baby.

How Does the Egg
Grow To Be a Baby?

First this fertilized egg divides into two parts.

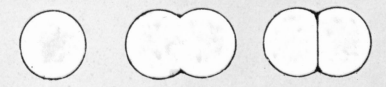

Then each of these two parts divides again, and all the parts continue to divide and divide and divide, though still attached together. This dividing is the way the egg grows.

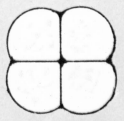

The first two months this little thing growing in the uterus doesn't look at all like a baby. But it doesn't look like a little round ball any more, either. It has started to change shape and develop.

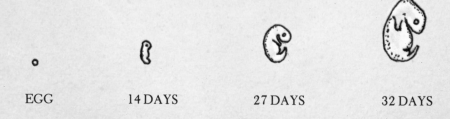

| EGG | 14 DAYS | 27 DAYS | 32 DAYS |

After the first two months it begins to look more like a baby, but it is still quite small—only about this size—

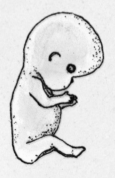

60 DAYS

But it grows and grows, and changes and changes, and gradually it looks more and more like a human baby—with mouth and eyes and nose and ears and arms and legs, and all the other parts of the body. At the end of about nine months a wonderful and exciting thing has happened: a fully formed baby is now ready to come out into the world.

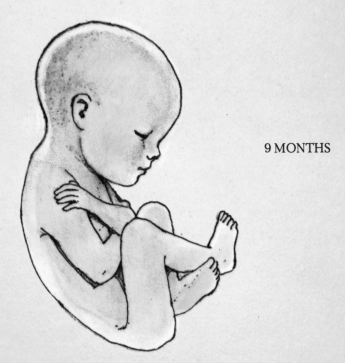

9 MONTHS

How Does the Baby
Live In the Uterus?

When a mother has a baby in her body, we say she is *pregnant*. As the baby is growing inside the uterus, the uterus is stretching and growing, too, giving the baby enough room.

While the baby is in the uterus, it is very well protected. It lies curled up inside a bag of fluid, or liquid, which keeps it from being bumped or hurt. The temperature inside the uterus is always warm and always the same. So the baby is really well taken care of during the nine months that it is inside its mother.

"But," you ask, "how does the baby eat and breathe inside the mother's body? And why doesn't the baby drown if it is in a bag of fluid?"

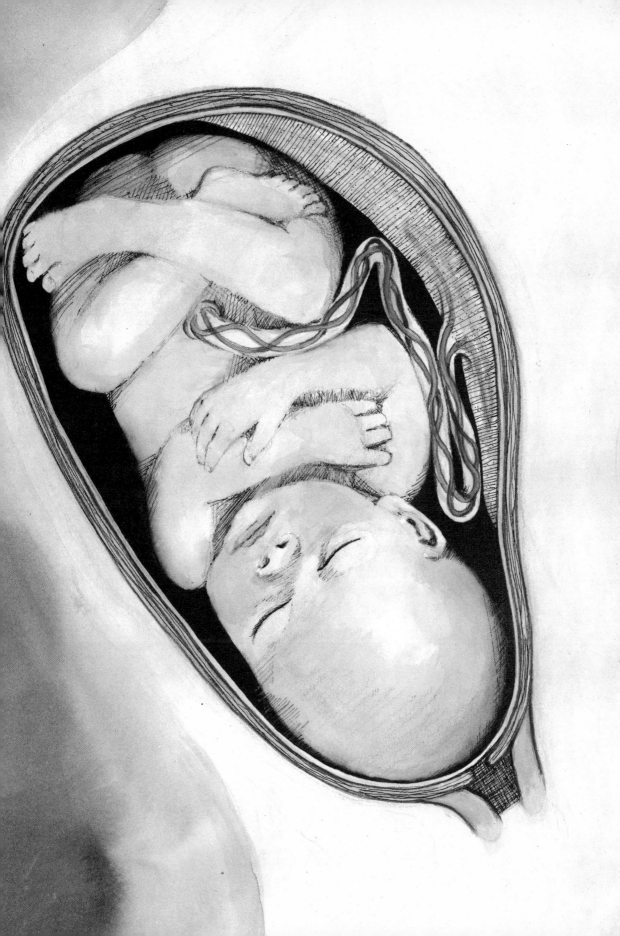

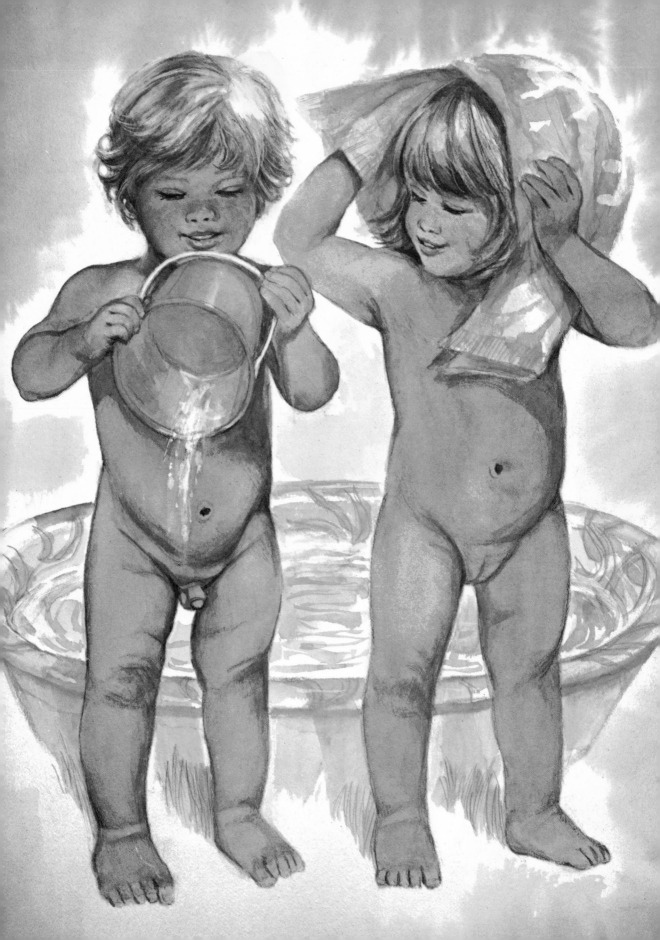

Now here is what may seem to be a strange answer. The baby, before it is born, does not eat with its mouth or breathe with its nose the way we do. We need food to eat, and air to breathe, in order to live and grow. But the unborn baby gets food and air from its mother's blood. This is how it happens.

Before a baby is born—while it is living inside its mother's body—it is attached to its mother by a *cord* containing three little tubes. One end of this cord is attached to the inside of the uterus of the mother. The other end is attached to the *navel* of the baby. (Do you know where the navel is? It is that round dented place on the outside of your body, which many people call the "belly button." Every person has a navel—every man, every woman, every boy, every girl.) The tubes inside the cord contain blood which carries food and air from the mother to the baby. It is not the kind of food that we eat, nor exactly the kind of air that we breathe, but a special kind of food and air that is in blood.

This is how the baby stays alive and grows inside of its mother. So you see that a pregnant mother is really keeping two people alive—she is eating and breathing for herself and also for her baby.

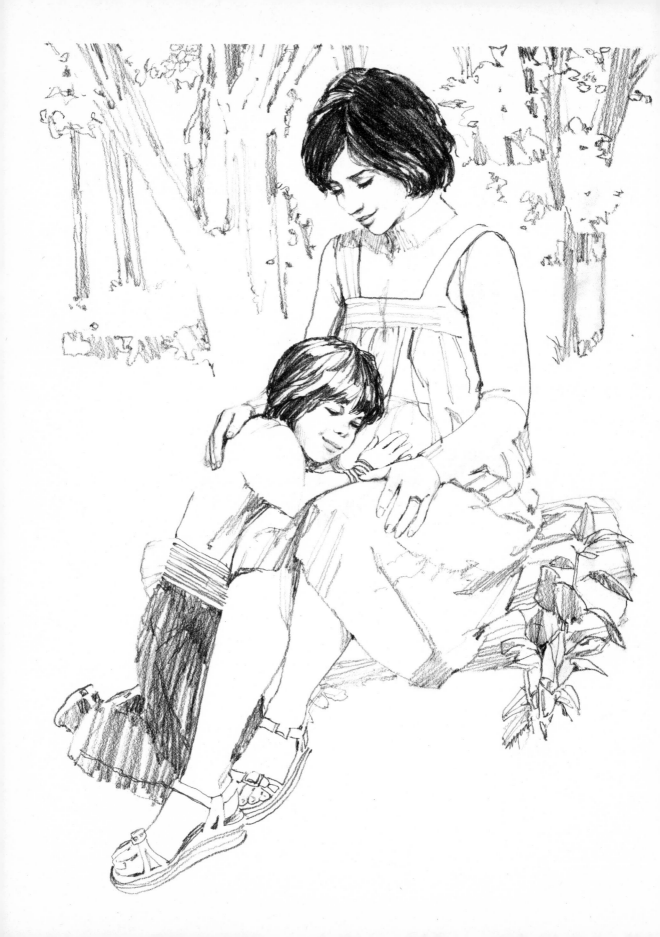

Can the Baby
Move In the Uterus?

During the first few months of its life inside the uterus the baby usually does not move. But after four or five months, it starts to move its arms and kick its feet, and even to turn around a bit. The mother can feel these little movements, too. They do not hurt her, of course, because the baby is so tiny that its kicks are quick, soft, and very gentle. In fact, the mother likes feeling these movements, because knowing that she is carrying a living child inside of her is very thrilling.

Usually a few weeks before the mother feels the baby's movements, the doctor can hear the baby's heart beat. He can hear it through his stethoscope—that instrument like a telephone that your doctor uses when he listens at your back or chest. He places his stethoscope on the outside of the mother's body over the uterus; he knows just where the right place is to hear the baby's heart beat. The baby's heart beats very quickly and sounds like the ticking of a watch under a pillow. When the doctor hears the heart beat, he knows that there is a living child in the mother's uterus.

How Is the Baby Born?

When nine months are over, the baby is fully formed and ready to leave the uterus to be born. Then the sides of the uterus begin to push in and out, squeezing down, harder and harder—until, at last, the baby is forced down and out of the mother's body through the vagina, the very same passage through which the sperm entered nine months before.

The head of the baby usually comes out first, stretching the vagina so that there is room enough for the body of the baby to follow.

The mother feels some pains when this is happening, but usually mothers do not mind these pains too much because they know that at the end of them their baby will be born. And having a baby is certainly worth a few pains.

Maybe you've been wondering how long it takes for a baby to be born. Usually it takes a few hours, but sometimes it takes only a few minutes, and occasionally it may take even a day or more.

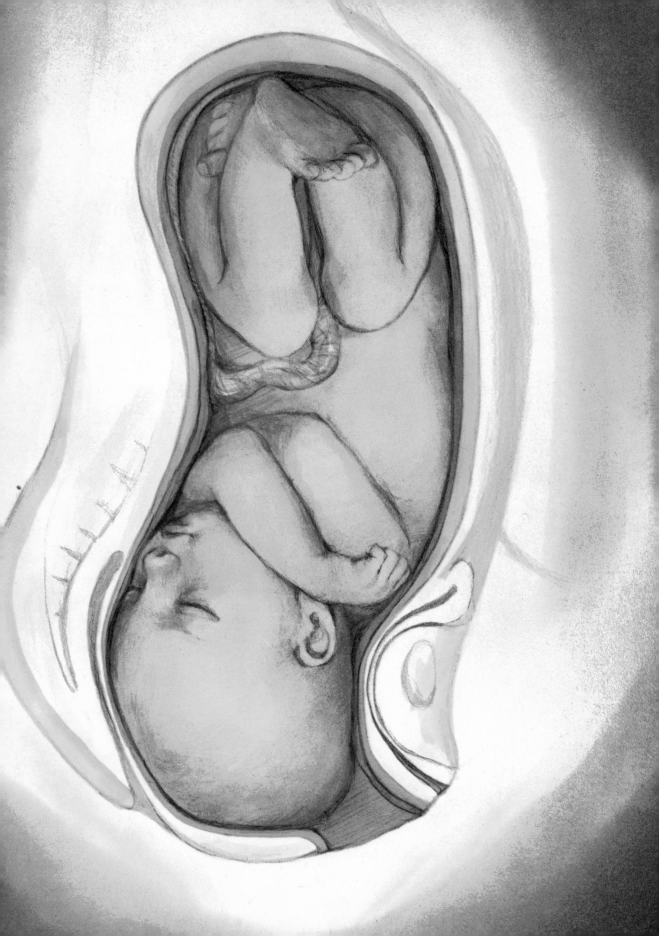

Almost at once after being born, a baby gives a little cry. That is the way all babies start breathing. From that time on they breathe all by themselves, both day and night, for the rest of their lives.

And that is how you were born.

After you were born, the doctor cut the cord which connected you to your mother. You were now out in the world at last. The cord which had brought you food and air was of no further use and so this cord, as well as the part that connected it to the uterus, was also forced out by the uterus.

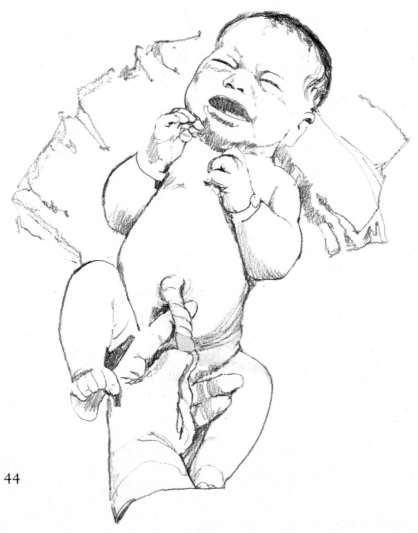

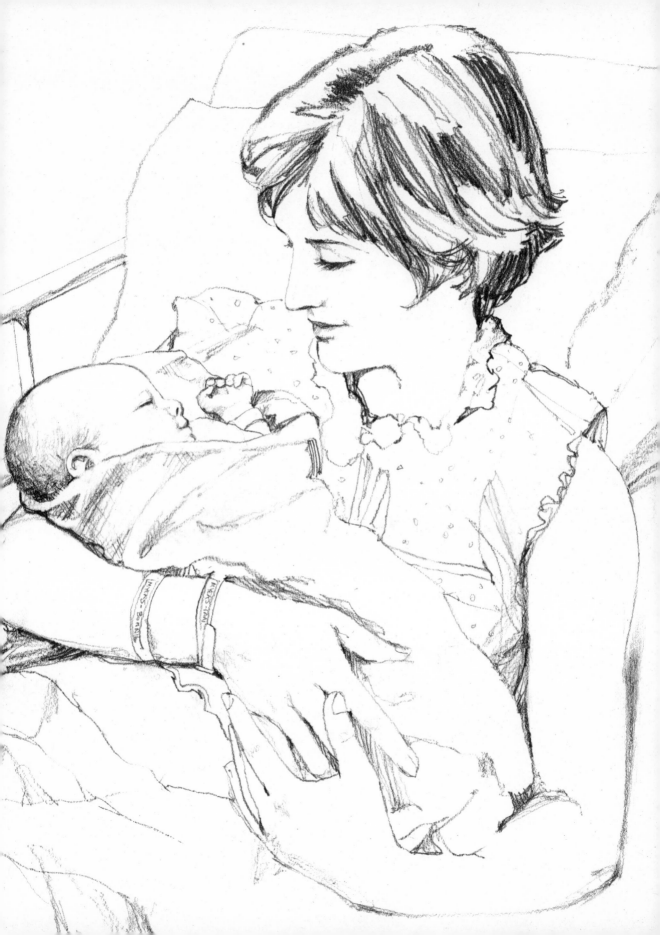

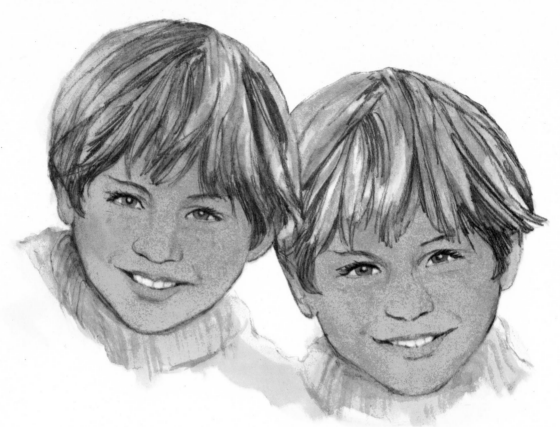

Twins, Triplets, and More

Sometimes mothers give birth to more than one baby at almost the same time. When two babies are born like this, they are called twins.

TWINS

You may be wondering about twins and how they come about.

Did you know that there are two kinds of twins? There are those that look almost exactly alike and they are called *identical twins*. Then there are twins that most often do not look alike and they are called *non-identical twins*.

46

Identical twins (one-egg twins)

Identical twins begin just the way a single baby does—from a single egg fertilized by a single sperm. You remember how the fertilized egg first divided into two parts, and divided and divided and divided until the whole baby was formed.

With identical twins something different happens. For some reason or other, when the egg first divides it splits right in two, making two separate eggs.

These two eggs are alike in every way and grow to form twin babies that look almost like one another. These identical twins are always the same sex—either two girls or two boys—and they will be born at almost the same time, one after the other.

Non-identical twins (two-egg twins)

Once in a while two eggs (instead of one) come out of the mother's ovary at about the same time. These two eggs are fertilized by two separate sperms— one sperm for one egg and one sperm for the other egg. Since each egg is different and each sperm is different, the two babies that are formed will be different.

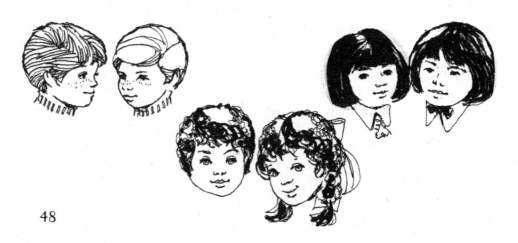

These two babies then grow and develop inside the mother's body just the way all babies do. And they will be born at almost the same time, one after the other, just like identical twins. But non-identical twins will not look any more alike than any two children born of the same mother and father. They may be the same sex—two boys or two girls—or different sexes—a boy and a girl.

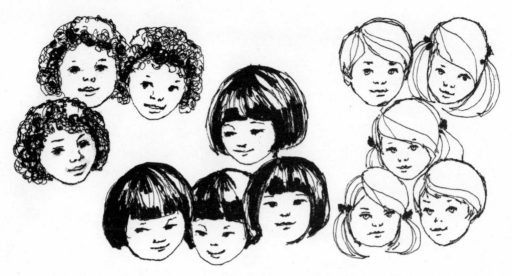

TRIPLETS, QUADRUPLETS, QUINTUPLETS.

When a mother gives birth to three babies at almost the same time, these babies are called *triplets*; four babies are called *quadruplets*; five babies are called *quintuplets*.

Triplets (three babies)

Triplets can be formed in a few different ways. They can come from three separate eggs, forming non-identical triplets:

Or they can come from two eggs, one of which splits to form twins, making one pair of identical twins and one single child.

Or they can come from one egg that divides and separates several times, forming identical triplets:

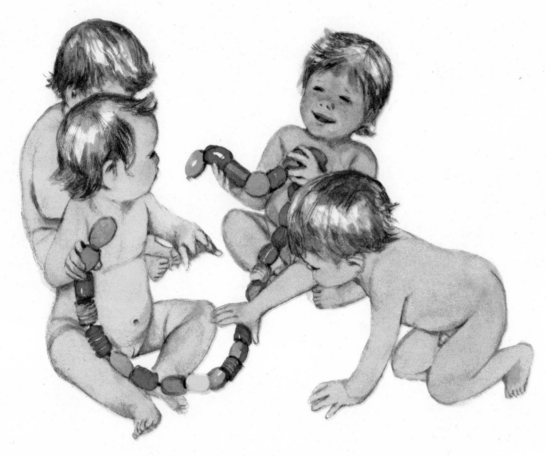

Quadruplets (four babies) and Quintuplets (five babies)

Quadruplets starting from 1 or 2 or 3 or 4 eggs and quintuplets starting from 1 or 2 or 3 or 4 or 5 eggs are formed in the same way. See if you can figure out all the different ways they may come about.

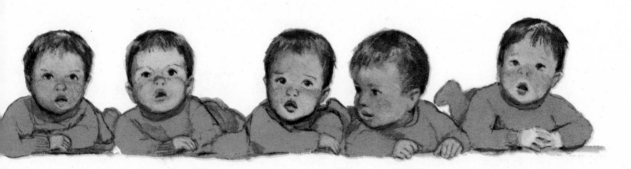

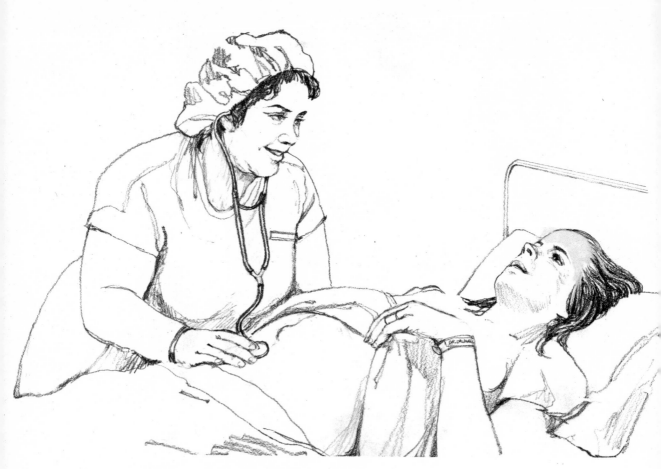

Why Are Most Babies Born in Hospitals?

Nowadays most, but not all, babies are born in hospitals. Mothers want to have a doctor to help make the birth of the baby easier and more comfortable. And doctors like to work in a hospital where everything is clean, where there are nurses to help, and where everything can be arranged to bring the most comfort and best care to the mother and to the baby. The mother can get a good rest while her new baby is being well taken care of.

Each baby has its own little crib to lie in, with its name on a white card attached to the crib. The baby's name is written on a bracelet around its wrist, or a necklace around its neck, so that everyone will know which parents it belongs to.

If a mother does not go to the hospital, she usually arranges for a doctor and a nurse, or a specially trained nurse called a midwife, to come to her home to help when the baby is born.

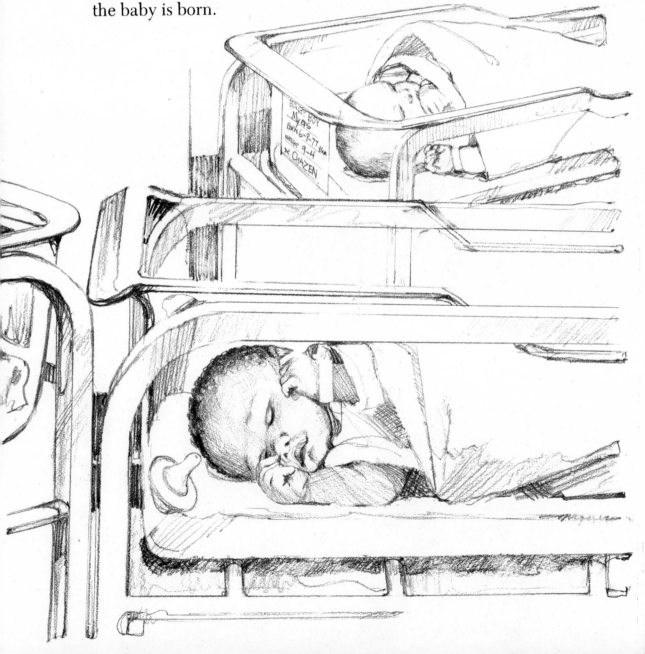

How Is the Newborn Baby Fed?

Before you were born, food had never entered your mouth. But as soon as you came out into the world, you were ready to be fed by mouth. When you were hungry, you started to make sucking movements with your lips the moment anything touched them. But you were just a little newborn baby and you couldn't get the food you needed all by yourself. So once again your mother gave you the food you needed.

Perhaps you drank milk from your mother's breasts, for they were ready for you when you needed them.

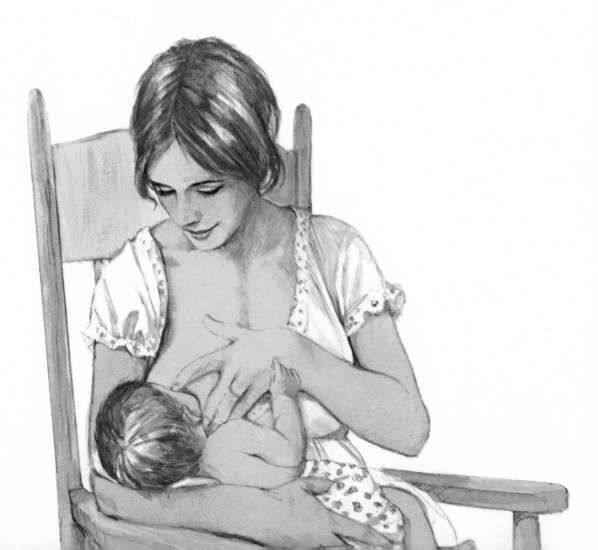

During the nine months when a baby grows inside the body of its mother, the mother's breasts are growing larger. But they do not have milk in them until after the baby is born. At this time the breasts start making milk. When the baby sucks on the breast, the milk begins to flow out. A baby does not have to be taught how to suck on the breast. It knows how to do it the minute it is born.

But not all mothers nurse their babies at the breast. Perhaps your mother fed you milk from a baby bottle when you were first born. This milk was just the right mixture, which made it very much like mother's milk.

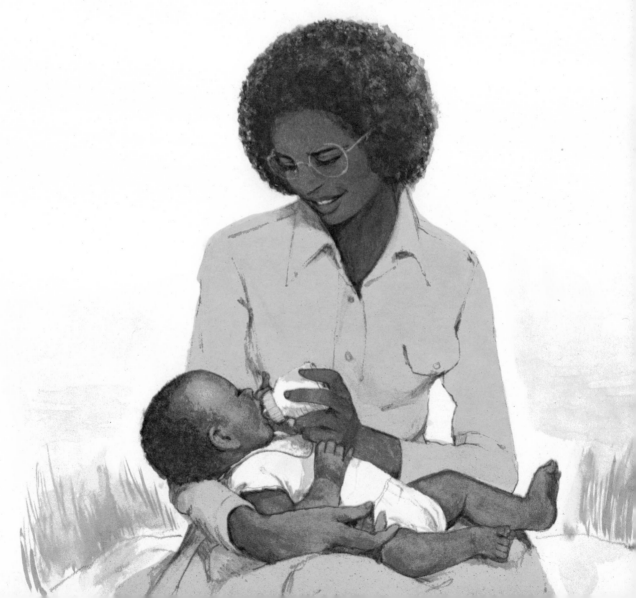

Growing Up

Just think how helpless you were when you were a newborn baby. You couldn't walk, you couldn't talk, you couldn't sit up, you couldn't even turn from one side to another.

You had no teeth. You could hardly see. You cried when you were hungry or uncomfortable or when you wanted to be held or hugged. Your mother had to feed you, and keep you clean, and keep you warm.

In a few weeks you were able to see better, and you started looking at things and watching people walk around.

When you were a new baby, you had many more meals than you have now. For the first few months you were probably fed every three or four hours during the day, and you may have been fed once or twice during the night also.

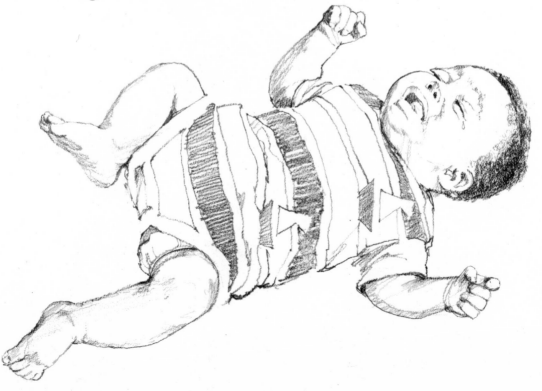

After a few months you were given a taste of cereal. Maybe you made a face at it or spit it out, for you had never had anything solid to eat before. But gradually you grew accustomed to cereal and then to other new foods—bananas, applesauce, prunes, carrots, spinach, peas—and one by one all the other fruits and vegetables, all strained and easy to eat because, you know, you were just beginning to get teeth.

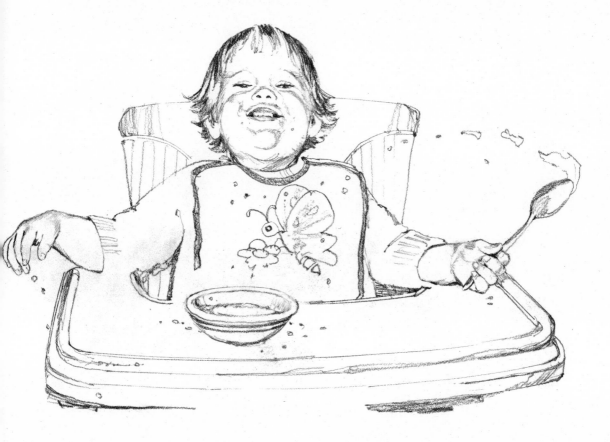

By the time you were a year old you were probably eating eggs and meat and fish too—and pretty soon you were eating almost everything that grown-up people eat.

And as you were growing, you began to do many things. You were able to sit up when you were about six months old.

You pulled yourself up when you were about nine months old.

You started walking by yourself when you were a little over a year old. And by the time you were two, you were, most likely, talking.

And you grew taller and you grew stronger. Now you were able to run and jump and play games.

And you are still growing, and will probably keep on growing until you are about twenty years old.

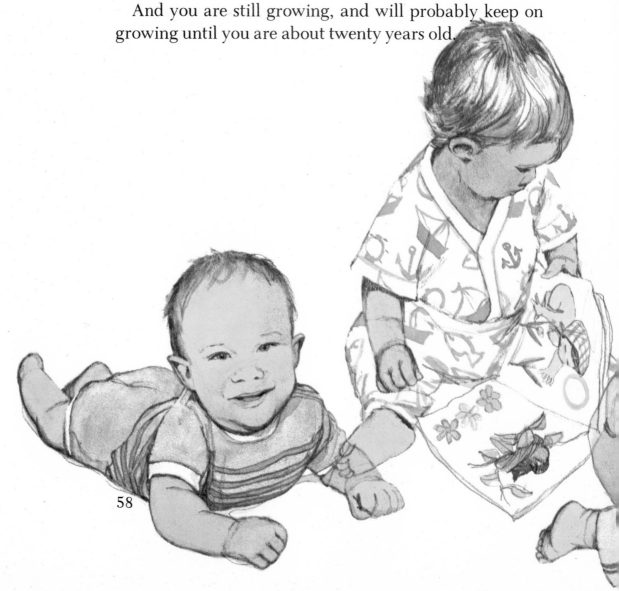

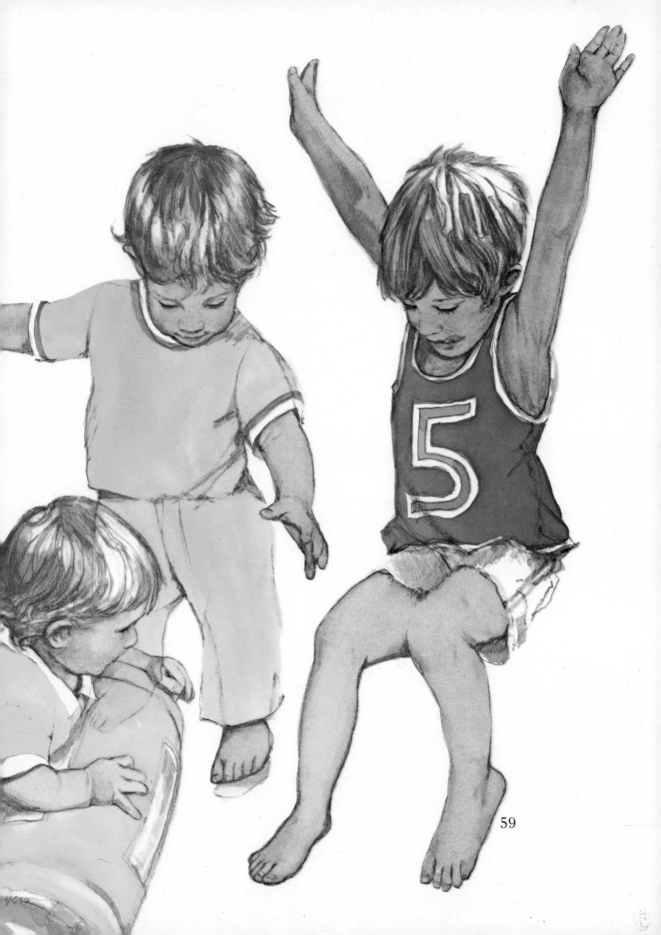

59

Boy to Man, Girl to Woman

After eleven or twelve or thirteen years of age, and up to about twenty years of age, there are changes in the bodies of boys and girls which gradually make them men and women.

In a girl, the breasts start to grow larger. Later, when she is fully grown, if she has a baby, her breasts will fill with milk so that she may be able to nurse it.

In a boy, the voice begins to get deeper, and beard and mustache hair starts to grow on his face.

During this time, also, the ovaries in girls begin to make eggs, while the testicles in boys start to make sperms.

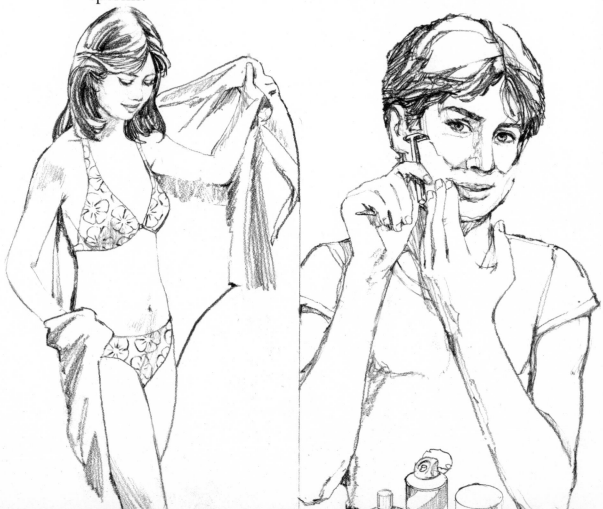

And so, when you are about twenty years old, you really will be grown up. You will be as tall as you ever will be, your muscles and bones will be fully grown, and you will be able to have children of your own.

The little newborn baby that once was you will have grown to be a man or a woman.

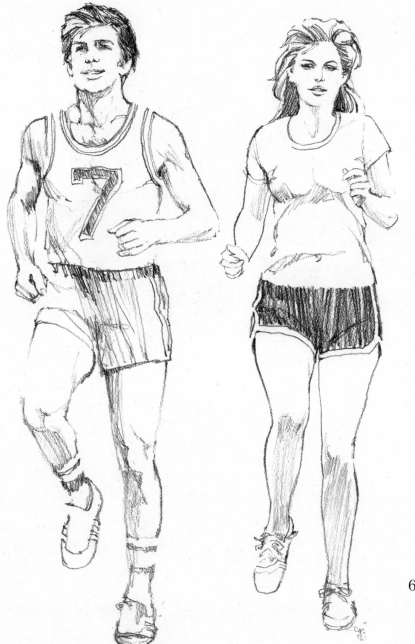

This story of starting life from a tiny egg, which was joined by a tiny sperm, of growing and developing in a warm and protected place inside the mother's body, and of being born, belongs to all human beings in the world. Every living person on earth began life in this way. It is your story, too, because this is the way that you began your life. It is your mother's and father's story, too, because they loved one another, and married, and made a home—and you came to be born because of their love.

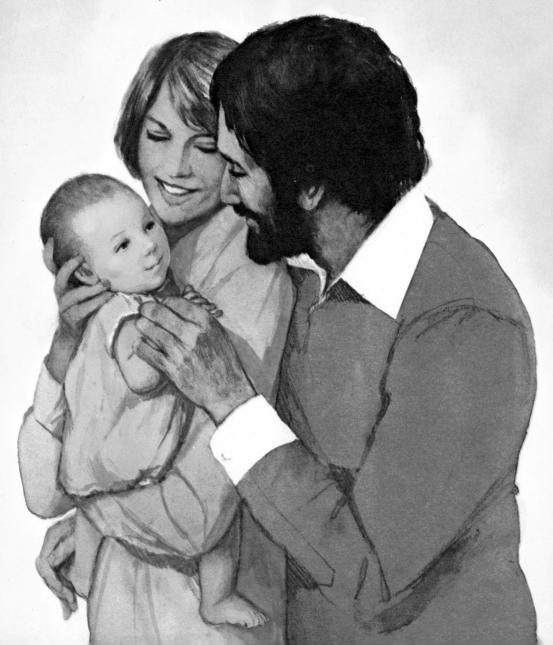

ABOUT THE AUTHORS

Milton I. Levine, M.D., and his wife, Jean H. Seligmann, are the parents of two children and live in New York City. Dr. Levine is a Clinical Professor of Pediatrics at Cornell University-New York Hospital Medical Center. He has been the pediatrician of the City and Country School in New York City since 1930 and for years held the same position at the Harriet Johnson Nursery School of Bank Street Schools in New York City. He is also a Consulting Pediatrician of the Bureau of Child Hygiene, New York City Department of Health. In addition, Dr. Levine is a Fellow of the American Academy of Pediatrics and the American Public Health Association.

Jean Seligmann specialized in psychology at Radcliffe College and is a graduate of the Froebel League Training School in New York City. She has been an assistant teacher at the Harriet Johnson Nursery School and at the City and Country School.

Both Dr. and Mrs. Levine are widely known authorities on the subject of child psychology and sex education. They are the authors of *The Wonder of Life*, a book on sex and reproduction written for older children, *The Parent's Encyclopedia*, and numerous magazine articles. Dr. Levine has also lectured frequently on television, radio and before parents' groups.

64

B C D E F